MUSCLE GAIN / WEIGHTLOSS

LOW CALORIE HIGH PROTEIN

MEAL PREP COOKBOOK

Attain optimal health, build muscle, and shed pounds with the ultimate high-protein regimen for a leaner, stronger, and thinner you!

Brittany Rice

TABLE OF CONTENT

INTRODUCTION

DO I NEED THIS COOKBOOK?

Welcome to a journey that harmonizes two remarkable goals—***building muscle and losing weight.*** This cookbook is a testament to the idea that achieving these ambitions is not mutually exclusive but rather complementary.

If you find yourself at the intersection of desiring a sculpted, stronger physique while also aiming to shed those extra pounds, this cookbook is designed precisely for you. It's a guiding light through the intricate yet rewarding path of combining muscle gain with weight loss—a harmony that requires balance, nourishment, and strategic meal planning.

Are you someone who's been torn between the pursuit of muscle definition and the desire to trim down? Have you struggled to find meals that cater to both objectives without compromising taste, satisfaction, or nutrition? If so, this cookbook serves as your solution.

Within these pages, you'll discover a treasure trove of recipes meticulously crafted to elevate your protein intake while managing caloric intake. Each dish is thoughtfully designed to fuel your muscles, facilitate recovery, and support fat loss—all without sacrificing flavor or variety.

Whether you're new to the world of fitness nutrition or a seasoned enthusiast seeking innovative culinary inspiration, this cookbook provides a roadmap. It's a compass guiding you toward meals that not only nourish your body but also align with your aspirations for a leaner, stronger, and healthier self.

Prepare to embark on a culinary adventure where taste and health converge. Embrace recipes that cater to your quest for muscle growth and weight management—a synergy that ensures you not only reach your fitness goals but exceed them.

CHAPTER 1: UNDERSTANDING MUSCLE GAIN AND WEIGHT LOSS

THE SCIENCE BEHIND MUSCLE GAIN AND WEIGHT LOSS

Achieving optimal body composition involves a delicate balance between two seemingly opposing goals: muscle gain and weight loss. Understanding the science behind these processes unveils the intricate mechanisms that drive transformations in our bodies.

Muscle Gain:

Building muscle relies on the concept of hypertrophy, the increase in muscle fiber size. This process occurs through mechanical tension (exercising with resistance), metabolic stress (muscles working under tension), and muscle damage (micro-tears repaired during recovery). Adequate protein intake, essential for repairing and growing muscle tissues, serves as a cornerstone in this process.

Weight Loss:

Weight loss, on the other hand, revolves around the principle of creating a caloric deficit. This means burning more calories than consumed. While the simplicity of this concept is clear, the mechanisms behind sustainable fat loss are multifaceted. Hormones, metabolic rate, and individual genetic factors play crucial roles.

The Intersection:

What's intriguing is the interplay between these seemingly contrasting goals. Often, weight loss may involve muscle loss, impacting metabolic rate and overall strength. However, through strategic nutrition and exercise, it's possible to promote fat loss while preserving or even increasing lean muscle mass.

Understanding the science behind muscle gain and weight loss empowers individuals to craft personalized approaches. Tailoring nutrition, exercise routines, and lifestyle choices based on these scientific principles can optimize results. Prioritizing high-protein, nutrient-dense foods, strategic resistance training, and a sustainable approach to calorie management can simultaneously support muscle gain and weight loss, leading to a healthier and more resilient body.

In essence, grasping this scientific foundation empowers individuals to navigate their fitness journey with informed decisions and targeted strategies, fostering not just physical change but also long-term health and wellness.

This understanding can serve as a guiding principle in crafting nutrition plans and exercise regimens for achieving both muscle gain and weight loss goals effectively.

BALANCING CALORIES FOR MUSCLE BUILDING AND FAT LOSS

Achieving the delicate equilibrium between calorie intake and expenditure is pivotal when pursuing both muscle building and fat loss. This process requires a strategic and nuanced approach to nutrition and exercise, emphasizing a balance that supports muscle growth while creating a caloric deficit for effective fat loss.

1. Establishing Caloric Goals:

- Determine your maintenance calories: Calculate the number of calories required to maintain your current weight.

- Create a surplus for muscle gain: Consume a slight caloric surplus to provide the energy necessary for muscle growth.

- Introduce a deficit for fat loss: Implement a modest caloric deficit to encourage the body to tap into stored fat for energy.

2. Prioritizing Protein Intake:

- Ensure an adequate protein intake to support muscle repair and growth.

- High-protein foods should be a cornerstone of your diet, helping preserve lean muscle mass during periods of caloric deficit.

3. Nutrient Timing:

- Optimize nutrient distribution throughout the day, with a focus on pre and post-workout nutrition.

- Prioritize protein and carbohydrates around workouts to fuel exercise performance and aid recovery.

4. Emphasizing Nutrient-Dense Foods:

- Choose nutrient-dense, whole foods to meet your caloric goals.

- Prioritize complex carbohydrates, lean proteins, and healthy fats to support overall health and performance.

5. Monitoring and Adjusting:

- Regularly assess progress and make adjustments to caloric intake based on changes in weight, muscle mass, and fat levels.

- Be adaptable to fluctuations and fine-tune your approach to meet evolving fitness goals.

6. Incorporating Resistance Training:

- Resistance training is crucial for muscle building; it not only expends calories during workouts but also contributes to an elevated metabolic rate post-exercise.

- Include a well-rounded strength training program to stimulate muscle growth and development.

7. Cardiovascular Exercise:

- Integrate cardiovascular activities strategically to enhance calorie expenditure and facilitate fat loss.

- Choose cardio exercises that complement your overall fitness plan without compromising muscle gains.

Balancing calories for muscle building and fat loss demands a personalized approach. It's essential to understand your body's unique requirements, track progress diligently, and make adjustments as needed. Remember, the key lies in finding the right equilibrium to promote both muscle development and sustainable fat loss over time.

IMPORTANCE OF HIGH PROTEIN AND LOW-CALORIE FOODS

In the pursuit of a balanced and effective approach to both muscle gain and weight loss, the significance of incorporating high protein and low-calorie foods cannot be overstated. These two nutritional components play distinct yet complementary roles in optimizing health and achieving fitness goals.

1. Muscle Building with High Protein:

Protein is the fundamental building block of muscles, making it indispensable for those seeking to enhance muscle mass. Consuming an ample amount of high-quality protein supports the repair and growth of muscle tissues, especially after intense physical activity. Whether you are engaged in resistance training or aiming to maintain existing muscle mass while losing weight, a protein-rich diet is key.

2. Weight Loss through Low-Calorie Foods:

Weight loss is fundamentally rooted in the principle of creating a calorie deficit—expending more calories than one consumes. Low-calorie foods play a crucial role in this process by allowing individuals to enjoy satisfying and nutritious meals without exceeding their daily caloric limits. By choosing nutrient-dense, low-calorie options, individuals can optimize their overall health while working towards their weight loss objectives.

3. Achieving Balance:

The synergy between high protein and low-calorie foods is the cornerstone of a balanced and sustainable nutrition strategy. Protein helps in preserving lean muscle mass during periods of calorie restriction, ensuring that weight loss primarily consists of fat rather than muscle tissue. Additionally, the satiating effect of protein-rich meals contributes to a feeling of fullness, aiding in appetite control and making it easier to adhere to a calorie-controlled diet.

4. Metabolic Benefits:

High protein intake has been linked to increased thermogenesis, meaning that the body expends more energy in the process of digesting and utilizing protein. This can contribute to a higher metabolic rate, potentially facilitating weight loss. Combining this metabolic advantage with the energy density of low-calorie foods creates a powerful strategy for achieving and maintaining a healthy weight.

In conclusion, the careful integration of high protein and low-calorie foods forms the foundation of a nutrition plan that supports both muscle gain and weight loss. This approach not only fosters physical well-being but also enhances the likelihood of long-term success by promoting sustainable dietary habits. Whether the goal is to sculpt a stronger physique, shed excess pounds, or achieve a harmonious balance of both, the combination of high protein and low-calorie foods is an invaluable asset on the journey to optimal health and fitness.

CHAPTER 2: MEAL PREP BASICS

GETTING STARTED WITH MEAL PREPPING

1. Understanding Meal Prepping:

Meal prepping involves planning, preparing, and packaging meals in advance. It allows for efficient use of time by cooking larger batches of food and portioning them out for future consumption.

2. Set Clear Objectives:

Define your goals for meal prepping. Whether it's saving time during the week, ensuring healthier eating habits, managing portion control, or sticking to a specific diet plan, having a clear purpose will guide your meal prep strategies.

3. Plan Your Meals:

Start by creating a meal plan for the week. Consider your nutritional needs, desired calorie intake, and balance of macronutrients. Choose recipes that align with your goals and are suitable for prepping in advance.

4. Stock Up on Supplies:

Invest in quality storage containers in various sizes to accommodate different portions. Additionally, having kitchen essentials like knives, cutting boards, foil, and cooking utensils simplifies the meal prepping process.

5. Choose Efficient Recipes:

Opt for recipes that are easy to prepare in bulk and can be stored without compromising taste or texture. Dishes that freeze well or can be refrigerated for several days are ideal for meal prepping.

6. Schedule a Prep Day:

Dedicate a specific day or time slot in your week for meal prepping. This allows you to focus solely on cooking, portioning, and storing your meals without interruptions.

7. Cook in Batches:

Prepare large quantities of proteins, grains, vegetables, and snacks at once. Batch cooking not only saves time but also ensures consistency and variety in your meals throughout the week.

8. Portion Control and Labeling:

Divide your prepared meals into individual portions using your storage containers. Label them with the date and contents to easily identify and track what you have in your fridge or freezer.

9. Store Properly:

Store your prepped meals in the refrigerator or freezer based on their shelf life. Proper storage helps maintain freshness and minimizes the risk of food spoilage.

10. Adapt and Evolve:

Be flexible and open to adjustments in your meal prepping routine. Experiment with new recipes, adapt portion sizes, and learn from your experience to refine your approach over time.

Mastering the basics of meal prepping lays the foundation for a more organized, nutritious, and stress-free approach to eating. By embracing this efficient method, you'll not only streamline your week but also foster healthier eating habits that align with your goals and lifestyle.

ESSENTIAL KITCHEN TOOLS AND EQUIPMENT

1. Food Storage Containers:

Investing in a variety of food storage containers in different sizes and shapes is fundamental. Opt for durable, airtight containers that are microwave and freezer-safe. These containers not only keep your meals fresh but also allow for easy portion control and convenient grab-and-go meals.

2. Meal Prep Containers:

Specifically designed meal prep containers with divided compartments are incredibly helpful. They enable you to organize different food groups or components of a meal, keeping them separate until ready to eat. These containers are excellent for creating balanced, pre-portioned meals.

3. Quality Knives and Cutting Boards:

A good set of sharp knives and reliable cutting boards are indispensable for efficient meal prep. Invest in a variety of knives suited for different tasks (chef's knife, paring knife, serrated knife) to ensure smooth slicing, dicing, and chopping. Opt for high-quality cutting boards that are easy to clean and maintain.

4. Kitchen Appliances:

While not essential, certain kitchen appliances can significantly expedite meal prep. A slow cooker, Instant Pot, blender, food processor, and microwave are incredibly useful tools for preparing meals in bulk, quickly cooking proteins, or creating smoothies and sauces.

5. Measuring Tools:

Accurate portioning is key in meal prep. Measuring cups, spoons, and a kitchen scale help ensure precise ingredient quantities, aiding in portion control and nutritional accuracy.

6. Cooking Utensils:

Stock your kitchen with essential cooking utensils like spatulas, mixing spoons, tongs, and ladles. Silicone utensils are particularly useful for non-stick cookware and are durable for long-term use.

7. Meal Planning Supplies:

Keep a collection of notepads, meal planners, and markers handy to jot down recipes, plan your meals for the week, and label your prepped containers with dates and contents.

8. Organization and Storage Solutions:

Maximize kitchen efficiency with organizational tools like shelf dividers, drawer organizers, and pantry containers. Having a well-organized kitchen facilitates easy access to ingredients, reducing prep time and stress.

By assembling these essential kitchen tools and equipment, you'll lay a solid foundation for successful and sustainable meal prep routines. These tools not only simplify the process but also empower you to take control of your nutrition, allowing you to create delicious, balanced meals tailored to your specific health and fitness goals.

PLANNING FOR SUCCESS: MEAL PREP TIPS AND TRICKS

1. Set Clear Goals:

Clearly define your dietary goals, whether it's weight loss, muscle gain, or simply eating healthier. Tailor your meal prep to align with these objectives, selecting recipes and portion sizes accordingly.

2. Plan Your Menu:

Design a menu for the week that includes a variety of nutrients and flavors. Balance macronutrients (proteins, carbohydrates, and fats) while incorporating diverse ingredients to prevent taste fatigue.

3. Create a Shopping List:

Once the menu is set, compile a comprehensive shopping list. Stick to the list while shopping to avoid impulse purchases and ensure you have all necessary ingredients for the week ahead.

4. Choose Versatile Recipes:

Opt for recipes that can be easily batch-cooked and portioned. Dishes that can be customized with different sauces, seasonings, or toppings add variety to meals throughout the week.

5. Invest in Proper Containers:

Invest in quality, airtight containers that are suitable for storing and reheating meals. Ensure they are microwave and dishwasher-safe for convenience.

6. Prep in Batches:

Dedicate a specific day or time slot each week for meal prep. Cook in bulk, preparing multiple meals simultaneously to save time and streamline the process.

7. Use Time-Saving Techniques:

Employ time-saving techniques like using a slow cooker, instant pot, or sheet pan meals to simplify cooking. Pre-chop vegetables, marinate proteins, or pre-cook grains for quicker assembly.

8. Portion Control:

Portion meals appropriately to align with your nutritional goals. Use measuring tools or portion control containers to ensure consistency and avoid overeating.

9. Store and Label Efficiently:

Once meals are prepared, store them in labeled containers, noting the date of preparation and meal contents. This ensures easy identification and helps in maintaining freshness.

10. Stay Flexible:

Be flexible with your meal prep routine. Life can be unpredictable, so adapt your plan if needed. Have backup options or emergency meals for unforeseen situations.

11. Consistency is Key:

Consistency is crucial for success. Make meal prepping a habit, and over time, it will become second nature, supporting your overall health and fitness goals.

CHAPTER 3: BREAKFASTS FOR MUSCLE GAIN AND WEIGHT LOSS

ENERGIZING BREAKFAST OPTIONS

Protein-Packed Egg White Omelette

Prep & Cooking Time:

15 minutes

Nutritional Info: (per serving)

Calories: 120

Protein: 20g

Carbohydrates: 5g

Fat: 2g

Ingredients:

- 4 egg whites

- 1 cup spinach (chopped)

- 1/4 cup diced tomatoes

- 1/4 cup diced bell peppers

- 2 tablespoons diced onions

- Salt and pepper to taste

- 1 teaspoon olive oil

Instructions:

1. In a bowl, whisk the egg whites until frothy and season with salt and pepper.

2. Heat olive oil in a non-stick skillet over medium heat.

3. Add onions and bell peppers, sauté until slightly tender.

4. Add spinach and tomatoes, cook until spinach wilts.

5. Pour the egg whites over the vegetables, tilt the pan to spread evenly.

6. Cook until the edges set, then fold the omelette in half.

7. Cook for another minute until the center is cooked through.

8. Serve hot.

Greek Yogurt Parfait

Prep & Cooking Time:

5 minutes

Nutritional Info: (per serving)

Calories: 220

Protein: 20g

Carbohydrates: 30g

Fat: 4g

Ingredients:

- 1 cup plain Greek yogurt

- 1/2 cup mixed berries (strawberries, blueberries, raspberries)

- 2 tablespoons granola

- 1 tablespoon honey or agave syrup (optional)

Instructions:

1. In a glass or bowl, layer Greek yogurt.

2. Add a layer of mixed berries on top.

3. Sprinkle granola over the berries.

4. Drizzle honey or agave syrup if desired.

5. Repeat layers if using a larger container.

6. Serve chilled.

High-Protein Banana Pancakes

Prep & Cooking Time:

10 minutes

Nutritional Info: (per serving - makes 2 servings)

Calories: 220

Protein: 12g

Carbohydrates: 25g

Fat: 8g

Ingredients:

- 1 ripe banana (mashed)

- 2 eggs

- 1/4 teaspoon cinnamon

- Cooking spray or coconut oil (for greasing)

Instructions:

1. In a bowl, mash the banana until smooth.

2. Add eggs and cinnamon, whisk until well combined.

3. Heat a non-stick skillet over medium heat and grease lightly.

4. Pour small portions of the batter onto the skillet.

5. Cook until bubbles form, then flip and cook the other side.

6. Repeat until all batter is used.

7. Serve warm.

Turkey and Vegetable Breakfast Wrap

Prep & Cooking Time:

15 minutes

Nutritional Info: (per serving - makes 2 servings)

Calories: 250

Protein: 20g

Carbohydrates: 25g

Fat: 8g

Ingredients:

- 2 whole wheat or spinach tortillas

- 4 slices turkey breast

- 1/2 cup chopped bell peppers

- 1/4 cup chopped onions

- 1/4 cup shredded low-fat cheese

- Salt and pepper to taste

- Cooking spray

Instructions:

1. Heat a skillet over medium heat and lightly spray with cooking spray.

2. Add onions and bell peppers, sauté until tender.

3. Push vegetables to the side and lay turkey slices in the skillet to warm.

4. Sprinkle shredded cheese on top of the turkey.

5. Once cheese melts, place the tortilla on top to warm it up.

6. Spoon the turkey and vegetable mix onto the tortilla.

7. Season with salt and pepper, then wrap tightly.

8. Serve warm.

Quinoa Breakfast Bowl

Prep & Cooking Time: 10 minutes (assuming quinoa is pre-cooked)

Nutritional Info: (per serving)

Calories: 280

Protein: 10g

Carbohydrates: 35g

Fat: 12g

Ingredients:

- 1/2 cup cooked quinoa

- 1/4 cup sliced almonds

- 1/2 cup mixed berries (blueberries, raspberries)

- 1 tablespoon honey or maple syrup

- 1/2 cup unsweetened almond milk (or milk of choice)

Instructions:

1. In a bowl, layer cooked quinoa.

2. Top with sliced almonds and mixed berries.

3. Drizzle honey or maple syrup over the bowl.

4. Pour almond milk over the mixture.

5. Mix well before eating.

PROTEIN-PACKED MORNING MEALS

Spinach and Feta Egg Muffins

Prep and Cooking Time:

30 minutes

Nutritional Info (per serving):

- Calories: 120

- Protein: 10g

- Carbohydrates: 2g

- Fat: 8g

Ingredients:

- 8 large eggs

- 1 cup baby spinach, chopped

- 1/2 cup feta cheese, crumbled

- 1/4 cup red bell pepper, diced

- Salt and pepper to taste

Instructions:

1. Preheat the oven to 350°F (175°C).

2. In a bowl, whisk the eggs and season with salt and pepper.

3. Stir in chopped spinach, feta cheese, and diced red bell pepper.

4. Grease a muffin tin and pour the egg mixture evenly into each cup.

5. Bake for 20-25 minutes or until the eggs are set.

6. Allow to cool, then store in airtight containers in the refrigerator.

Greek Yogurt Parfait with Berries and Almonds

Prep Time:

5 minutes

Nutritional Info (per serving):

- Calories: 250

- Protein: 20g

- Carbohydrates: 20g

- Fat: 10g

Ingredients:

- 1 cup Greek yogurt

- 1/2 cup mixed berries (blueberries, strawberries, raspberries)

- 2 tablespoons almonds, chopped

- 1 tablespoon honey

Instructions:

1. In a glass or jar, layer Greek yogurt, mixed berries, and chopped almonds.

2. Drizzle honey on top.

3. Repeat the layers.

4. Seal the container and store in the refrigerator.

Quinoa Breakfast Bowl with Cottage Cheese and Nuts

Prep Time:

10 minutes

Nutritional Info (per serving):

- Calories: 320

- Protein: 25g

- Carbohydrates: 25g

- Fat: 15g

Ingredients:

- 1/2 cup cooked quinoa

- 1/2 cup low-fat cottage cheese

- 1/4 cup mixed nuts (almonds, walnuts, pistachios)

- 1 tablespoon chia seeds

- 1/2 teaspoon cinnamon

Instructions:

1. In a bowl, combine cooked quinoa and cottage cheese.

2. Top with mixed nuts, chia seeds, and a sprinkle of cinnamon.

3. Mix well and refrigerate in a sealed container.

Protein-Packed Banana Pancakes

Prep and Cooking Time:

15 minutes

Nutritional Info (per serving):

- Calories: 280

- Protein: 25g

- Carbohydrates: 30g

- Fat: 8g

Ingredients:

- 1 ripe banana, mashed

- 2 eggs

- 1/4 cup protein powder (vanilla or chocolate)

- 1/2 teaspoon baking powder

- 1/2 teaspoon vanilla extract

Instructions:

1. In a bowl, combine mashed banana, eggs, protein powder, baking powder, and vanilla extract.

2. Mix until smooth.

3. Heat a non-stick skillet over medium heat and pour 1/4 cup of batter for each pancake.

4. Cook until bubbles form on the surface, then flip and cook the other side.

5. Stack pancakes and store in an airtight container.

Turkey and Vegetable Breakfast Burritos

Prep and Cooking Time:

20 minutes

Nutritional Info (per serving):

- Calories: 350

- Protein: 30g

- Carbohydrates: 25g

- Fat: 15g

Ingredients:

- 4 whole-grain tortillas

- 8 large eggs, scrambled

- 1 cup lean ground turkey, cooked

- 1/2 cup black beans, drained and rinsed

- 1/4 cup low-fat shredded cheese

- Salsa for topping

Instructions:

1. In each tortilla, layer scrambled eggs, ground turkey, black beans, and shredded cheese.

2. Roll up the burritos, folding in the edges.

3. Wrap each burrito in foil and store in the refrigerator.

SUPER LOW CALORIE BREAKFAST IDEAS FOR WEIGHT LOSS

Egg White and Spinach Omelette

Prep/Cook Time:

10 minutes

Nutritional Info:

Calories: 120

Protein: 20g

Carbohydrates: 4g

Fat: 3g

Ingredients:

- 4 egg whites
- 1 cup fresh spinach, chopped
- 1/4 cup diced tomatoes
- 2 tablespoons diced onion
- Salt and pepper to taste
- 1 teaspoon olive oil

Instructions:

1. Heat olive oil in a non-stick skillet over medium heat.

2. Sauté onions until translucent, then add spinach and tomatoes. Cook until spinach wilts.

3. In a bowl, whisk egg whites and season with salt and pepper.

4. Pour the egg mixture into the skillet, swirling to spread evenly.

5. Cook for 2-3 minutes until the edges start to set, then fold the omelette in half.

6. Cook for another minute or until eggs are fully cooked.

7. Serve hot.

Greek Yogurt Parfait

Prep/Cook Time:

5 minutes

Nutritional Info:

Calories: 200 | Protein: 20g | Carbohydrates: 20g | Fat: 6g

Ingredients:

- 1 cup Greek yogurt (unsweetened)
- 1/2 cup mixed berries (strawberries, blueberries, raspberries)
- 2 tablespoons chopped almonds
- 1 teaspoon honey (optional)

Instructions:

1. In a glass or bowl, layer Greek yogurt, mixed berries, and chopped almonds.
2. Drizzle with honey if desired.
3. Serve chilled.

Protein-Packed Chia Seed Pudding

Prep/Cook Time:

5 minutes (plus chilling time)

Nutritional Info:

Calories: 180 | Protein: 15g | Carbohydrates: 12g | Fat: 8g

Ingredients:

- 2 tablespoons chia seeds

- 1 cup unsweetened almond milk

- 1/2 scoop vanilla protein powder

- 1/2 teaspoon vanilla extract

- Stevia or sweetener of choice (optional)

- Fresh berries for topping

Instructions:

1. In a bowl, mix chia seeds, almond milk, protein powder, vanilla extract, and sweetener (if using).

2. Whisk well and let it sit for 5 minutes, then whisk again to prevent clumping.

3. Refrigerate overnight or for at least 3 hours until the mixture thickens.

4. Top with fresh berries before serving.

Turkey and Veggie Breakfast Wrap

Prep/Cook Time:

10 minutes

Nutritional Info:

Calories: 180

Protein: 20g

Carbohydrates: 8g

Fat: 7g

Ingredients:

- 2 large lettuce leaves or whole-grain wraps

- 3 slices turkey breast

- 1/4 cup diced bell peppers

- 1/4 cup diced cucumber

- 2 tablespoons hummus

- Fresh herbs (parsley or cilantro, optional)

Instructions:

1. Lay lettuce leaves or wraps flat on a clean surface.

2. Spread hummus on each wrap.

3. Layer turkey slices, diced bell peppers, and cucumber.

4. Add fresh herbs if desired.

5. Roll tightly and slice in half.

Quinoa and Cottage Cheese Breakfast Bowl

Prep/Cook Time:

5 minutes

Nutritional Info:

Calories: 250

Protein: 20g

Carbohydrates: 30g

Fat: 6g

Ingredients:

- 1/2 cup cooked quinoa

- 1/2 cup low-fat cottage cheese

- 1 tablespoon chopped nuts (walnuts, almonds)

- 1/4 cup diced mixed fruits (apple, banana, berries)

- Cinnamon powder for sprinkling

Instructions:

1. In a bowl, layer cooked quinoa and cottage cheese.

2. Top with diced fruits and chopped nuts.

3. Sprinkle with cinnamon powder for added flavor.

CHAPTER 4: LUNCHES FOR BUILDING MUSCLE AND LOSING WEIGHT

BALANCED LUNCH RECIPES

Grilled Chicken Quinoa Salad Bowl

Prep and Cooking Time:

30 minutes

Nutritional Info (per serving):

- Calories: 400

- Protein: 35g

- Carbohydrates: 30g

- Fat: 15g

Ingredients:

- 8 oz boneless, skinless chicken breast

- 1 cup quinoa (uncooked)

- 2 cups mixed salad greens

- 1 cup cherry tomatoes, halved

- 1 cucumber, diced

- 1/4 cup feta cheese, crumbled

- 2 tbsp olive oil

- 1 lemon, juiced

- Salt and pepper to taste

Instructions:

1. Cook quinoa according to package instructions.

2. Season chicken with salt and pepper, then grill until fully cooked.

3. In a large bowl, combine cooked quinoa, salad greens, cherry tomatoes, cucumber, and feta cheese.

4. Slice grilled chicken and place on top of the salad.

5. In a small bowl, whisk together olive oil, lemon juice, salt, and pepper to create the dressing.

6. Drizzle the dressing over the salad and toss gently to combine.

Lentil and Vegetable Stir-Fry with Tofu

Prep and Cooking Time:

25 minutes

Nutritional Info (per serving):

- Calories: 380

- Protein: 30g

- Carbohydrates: 45g

- Fat: 12g

Ingredients:

- 1 cup dry green lentils

- 14 oz firm tofu, cubed

- 2 cups broccoli florets

- 1 red bell pepper, sliced

- 1 carrot, julienned

- 3 tbsp low-sodium soy sauce

- 1 tbsp sesame oil

- 2 cloves garlic, minced

- 1 tsp ginger, grated

Instructions:

1. Cook lentils according to package instructions.

2. In a large wok or skillet, heat sesame oil over medium heat.

3. Add tofu cubes and stir-fry until golden brown.

4. Add garlic and ginger to the tofu, followed by broccoli, bell pepper, and carrot. Stir-fry until vegetables are tender-crisp.

5. Add cooked lentils and soy sauce, tossing everything together until well combined.

Turkey and Quinoa Stuffed Bell Peppers

Prep and Cooking Time:

40 minutes

Nutritional Info (per serving):

- Calories: 420

- Protein: 35g

- Carbohydrates: 40g

- Fat: 15g

Ingredients:

- 4 large bell peppers, halved and seeds removed
- 1 lb ground turkey
- 1 cup quinoa, cooked
- 1 can (15 oz) black beans, drained and rinsed
- 1 cup corn kernels
- 1 cup salsa
- 1 tsp cumin
- 1 tsp chili powder
- Salt and pepper to taste
- 1 cup shredded low-fat cheddar cheese

Instructions:

1. Preheat the oven to 375°F (190°C).
2. In a skillet, cook ground turkey until browned. Drain excess fat.
3. In a large bowl, combine cooked turkey, quinoa, black beans, corn, salsa, cumin, chili powder, salt, and pepper.
4. Stuff each bell pepper half with the turkey-quinoa mixture.
5. Top each stuffed pepper with shredded cheddar cheese.
6. Bake in the preheated oven for 20-25 minutes or until peppers are tender.

Salmon and Asparagus Foil Packets

Prep and Cooking Time:

25 minutes

Nutritional Info (per serving):

- Calories: 380

- Protein: 35g

- Carbohydrates: 10g

- Fat: 22g

Ingredients:

- 4 salmon fillets (6 oz each)

- 1 lb asparagus, trimmed

- 2 tbsp olive oil

- 4 cloves garlic, minced

- 1 lemon, sliced

- Fresh dill for garnish

- Salt and pepper to taste

Instructions:

1. Preheat the oven to 400°F (200°C).

2. Place each salmon fillet on a piece of aluminum foil.

3. Arrange asparagus around the salmon.

4. Drizzle olive oil over salmon and asparagus. Sprinkle minced garlic, salt, and pepper.

5. Top each salmon fillet with lemon slices and fresh dill.

6. Fold the foil to create sealed packets and bake in the preheated oven for 20 minutes.

Shrimp and Vegetable Stir-Fry with Brown Rice

Prep and Cooking Time:

30 minutes

Nutritional Info (per serving):

- Calories: 420

- Protein: 30g

- Carbohydrates: 60g

- Fat: 8g

Ingredients:

- 1 lb large shrimp, peeled and deveined

- 2 cups broccoli florets

- 1 red bell pepper, sliced

- 1 cup snap peas

- 3 cups cooked brown rice

- 3 tbsp low-sodium soy sauce

- 1 tbsp honey

- 1 tbsp sesame oil

- 2 cloves garlic, minced

- 1 tsp ginger, grated

- Green onions for garnish

Instructions:

1. In a bowl, whisk together soy sauce, honey, sesame oil, garlic, and ginger to make the sauce.

2. In a large skillet, cook shrimp until pink and opaque. Remove from the skillet and set aside.

3. Stir-fry broccoli, bell pepper, and snap peas in the same skillet until crisp-tender.

4. Add cooked shrimp back to the skillet, along with the sauce. Toss until everything is well coated.

5. Serve the shrimp and vegetable stir-fry over cooked brown rice, garnished with green onions.

HIGH-PROTEIN LUNCH FOR MUSCLE-GAIN

Grilled Chicken Quinoa Salad

Prep and Cooking Time:

30 minutes

Nutritional Info (per serving):

Calories: 380

Protein: 30g

Carbohydrates: 30g

Fat: 15g

Fiber: 4g

Ingredients:

- 2 boneless, skinless chicken breasts

- 1 cup quinoa

- 2 cups mixed greens

- 1 cup cherry tomatoes, halved

- 1 cucumber, diced

- 1/4 cup red onion, finely chopped

- 1/4 cup feta cheese (optional)

- Olive oil

- Lemon juice

- Salt and pepper

Instructions:

1. Cook quinoa according to package instructions. Set aside to cool.

2. Season chicken breasts with salt, pepper, and a drizzle of olive oil. Grill until cooked through. Let them rest before slicing.

3. In a large bowl, mix mixed greens, cherry tomatoes, cucumber, red onion, and cooked quinoa.

4. Add sliced grilled chicken on top.

5. Drizzle with olive oil, lemon juice, salt, and pepper. Toss gently to combine.

6. Optional: Sprinkle with feta cheese.

Turkey and Veggie Lettuce Wraps

Prep and Cooking Time:

25 minutes

Nutritional Info (per serving, wrap filling only, excluding lettuce):

Calories: 220

Protein: 28g

Carbohydrates: 5g

Fat: 10g

Fiber: 1g

Ingredients:

- 1 pound lean ground turkey
- 1 tablespoon olive oil
- 1 bell pepper, diced
- 1 zucchini, diced
- 2 cloves garlic, minced
- 2 tablespoons low-sodium soy sauce
- 1 teaspoon ground ginger
- Lettuce leaves for wrapping

Instructions:

1. Heat olive oil in a skillet over medium heat. Add ground turkey and cook until browned.

2. Add bell pepper, zucchini, and garlic. Cook until vegetables are tender.

3. Stir in soy sauce and ground ginger. Cook for an additional 2-3 minutes.

4. Spoon the turkey and veggie mixture into lettuce leaves, creating wraps.

Tuna and White Bean Salad

Prep and Cooking Time:

15 minutes

Nutritional Info (per serving):*

Calories: 310

Protein: 35g

Carbohydrates: 25g

Fat: 9g

Fiber: 7g

Ingredients:

- 2 cans (5 oz each) of tuna, drained

- 1 can (15 oz) white beans, rinsed and drained

- 1 red bell pepper, diced

- 1/4 cup red onion, finely chopped

- 2 tablespoons chopped parsley

- 2 tablespoons olive oil

- 1 tablespoon red wine vinegar

- Salt and pepper to taste

Instructions:

1. In a large bowl, combine tuna, white beans, red bell pepper, red onion, and parsley.

2. Drizzle with olive oil and red wine vinegar. Toss gently to coat.

3. Season with salt and pepper according to taste.

Veggie-Packed Chicken Stir-Fry

Prep and Cooking Time:

25 minutes

Nutritional Info (per serving, without rice):

Calories: 280

Protein: 30g

Carbohydrates: 20g

Fat: 8g

Fiber: 5g

Ingredients:

- 2 boneless, skinless chicken breasts, diced

- 2 cups broccoli florets

- 1 bell pepper, sliced

- 1 cup snap peas

- 2 cloves garlic, minced

- 2 tablespoons low-sodium soy sauce

- 1 tablespoon sesame oil

- 1 tablespoon honey

- 1 teaspoon cornstarch (optional, for thicker sauce)

- Cooked brown rice (optional, for serving)

Instructions:

1. In a bowl, mix soy sauce, sesame oil, honey, and cornstarch (if using). Set aside.

2. In a large skillet or wok, cook diced chicken until browned. Remove from the skillet.

3. Stir-fry garlic, broccoli, bell pepper, and snap peas until tender-crisp.

4. Add the cooked chicken back to the skillet and pour the sauce over the mixture.

5. Cook for a few more minutes until the sauce thickens.

6. Serve over cooked brown rice if desired.

Lentil and Chickpea Salad Bowl

Prep and Cooking Time:

20 minutes (assuming lentils and chickpeas are pre-cooked)

Nutritional Info (per serving):

Calories: 320

Protein: 20g

Carbohydrates: 40g

Fat: 10g

Fiber: 12g

Ingredients:

- 1 cup cooked lentils

- 1 cup cooked chickpeas

- 1 cucumber, diced

- 1 cup cherry tomatoes, halved

- 1/4 cup red onion, finely chopped

- 2 tablespoons chopped fresh mint

- 2 tablespoons olive oil

- Juice of 1 lemon

- Salt and pepper to taste

Instructions:

1. In a large bowl, combine cooked lentils, chickpeas, cucumber, cherry tomatoes, red onion, and fresh mint.

2. Drizzle with olive oil and lemon juice. Toss gently to mix.

3. Season with salt and pepper according to taste.

Absolutely, here are five detailed lunch recipes that focus on muscle building while supporting weight loss goals:

Grilled Chicken Veggie Bowl

Prep/Cook Time:

25 minutes

Nutritional Info (per serving):

- Calories: 320

- Protein: 35g

- Carbohydrates: 12g

- Fat: 14g

Ingredients:

- 2 boneless, skinless chicken breasts

- 1 tablespoon olive oil

- 2 cups broccoli florets

- 1 red bell pepper, sliced

- 1 yellow bell pepper, sliced

- 1 tablespoon balsamic vinegar

- Salt and pepper to taste

Instructions:

1. Preheat grill to medium-high heat.

2. Season chicken breasts with salt, pepper, and a drizzle of olive oil. Grill for 6-7 minutes per side or until cooked through.

3. Toss broccoli and bell peppers with olive oil, balsamic vinegar, salt, and pepper. Grill in a vegetable basket for 8-10 minutes until tender.

4. Divide grilled chicken and veggies into meal prep containers.

Quinoa and Black Bean Salad

Prep/Cook Time:

15 minutes

Nutritional Info (per serving):

- Calories: 280

- Protein: 14g

- Carbohydrates: 42g

- Fat: 7g

Ingredients:

- 1 cup cooked quinoa

- 1 can black beans, drained and rinsed

- 1 cup cherry tomatoes, halved

- 1/4 cup red onion, finely chopped

- 1/4 cup cilantro, chopped

- Juice of 1 lime

- 1 tablespoon olive oil

- Salt and pepper to taste

Instructions:

1. In a large bowl, mix cooked quinoa, black beans, cherry tomatoes, red onion, and cilantro.

2. Drizzle with olive oil and lime juice. Season with salt and pepper. Mix well.

3. Portion into meal prep containers.

Turkey and Spinach Stuffed Peppers

Prep/Cook Time:

50 minutes

Nutritional Info (per serving):

- Calories: 290

- Protein: 27g

- Carbohydrates: 26g

- Fat: 8g

Ingredients:

- 4 large bell peppers, halved and seeded

- 1 pound lean ground turkey

- 1 cup quinoa, cooked

- 2 cups spinach, chopped

- 1 can diced tomatoes, drained

- 1 teaspoon garlic powder

- 1 teaspoon paprika

- Salt and pepper to taste

Instructions:

1. Preheat oven to 375°F (190°C).

2. In a skillet, cook ground turkey until browned. Add spinach and cook until wilted. Stir in cooked quinoa, diced tomatoes, garlic powder, paprika, salt, and pepper.

3. Stuff the halved bell peppers with the turkey-quinoa mixture.

4. Place stuffed peppers in a baking dish. Cover with foil and bake for 25-30 minutes.

5. Allow to cool before portioning into meal prep containers.

Tuna and White Bean Salad

Prep/Cook Time:

15 minutes

Nutritional Info (per serving):

- Calories: 320

- Protein: 35g

- Carbohydrates: 29g

- Fat: 9g

Ingredients:

- 2 cans tuna, drained

- 2 cups white beans, cooked

- 1 cucumber, diced

- 1/4 cup red onion, finely chopped

- 2 tablespoons lemon juice

- 2 tablespoons olive oil

- 1 teaspoon Dijon mustard

- Salt and pepper to taste

Instructions:

1. In a large bowl, mix tuna, white beans, cucumber, and red onion.

2. In a separate bowl, whisk together lemon juice, olive oil, Dijon mustard, salt, and pepper.

3. Pour the dressing over the tuna and bean mixture. Toss until well combined.

4. Divide into meal prep containers.

Baked Salmon with Asparagus

Prep/Cook Time:

 20 minutes

Nutritional Info (per serving):

- Calories: 340

- Protein: 34g

- Carbohydrates: 6g

- Fat: 20g

Ingredients:

- 4 salmon fillets

- 1 tablespoon olive oil

- 2 cloves garlic, minced

- 1 teaspoon paprika

- 1 pound asparagus, trimmed

- Lemon wedges for serving

- Salt and pepper to taste

Instructions:

1. Preheat oven to 400°F (200°C).

2. Place salmon fillets on a baking sheet. Drizzle with olive oil and sprinkle minced garlic, paprika, salt, and pepper.

3. Arrange asparagus around the salmon. Drizzle with olive oil and season with salt and pepper.

4. Bake for 12-15 minutes until salmon is cooked through and asparagus is tender.

5. Allow to cool before dividing into meal prep containers.

CHAPTER 5: DINNERS TO SUPPORT MUSCLE GROWTH AND FAT LOSS

NUTRIENT-DENSE DINNER IDEAS

Grilled Lemon Herb Chicken with Roasted Vegetables

Prep/Cooking Time:

30-40 minutes

Nutritional Info: (Per Serving - Chicken and Vegetables)

- Calories: 280

- Protein: 35g

- Carbohydrates: 8g

- Fat: 12g

- Fiber: 3g

Ingredients:

- 4 boneless, skinless chicken breasts

- 2 tablespoons olive oil

- 2 cloves garlic, minced

- 1 teaspoon dried oregano

- 1 teaspoon dried thyme

- Juice of 1 lemon

- Salt and pepper to taste

- 2 cups mixed vegetables (zucchini, bell peppers, cherry tomatoes)

- Cooking spray

Instructions:

1. Preheat the grill to medium-high heat.

2. In a bowl, mix olive oil, garlic, oregano, thyme, lemon juice, salt, and pepper. Marinate chicken breasts in this mixture for 15-20 minutes.

3. Place marinated chicken on the grill and cook for 6-8 minutes per side until fully cooked.

4. Toss mixed vegetables with olive oil, salt, and pepper. Spread them on a baking sheet lined with parchment paper and roast in the oven at 400°F (200°C) for 15-20 minutes or until tender.

5. Serve grilled chicken alongside roasted vegetables.

Baked Salmon with Quinoa and Steamed Broccoli

Prep/Cooking Time:

30-35 minutes

Nutritional Info: (Per Serving - Salmon, Quinoa, and Broccoli)

- Calories: 320

- Protein: 28g

- Carbohydrates: 20g

- Fat: 15g

- Fiber: 5g

Ingredients:

- 4 salmon fillets

- 1 tablespoon olive oil

- 2 tablespoons lemon juice

- 1 teaspoon paprika

- Salt and pepper to taste

- 1 cup quinoa, rinsed

- 2 cups water or low-sodium broth

- 2 cups broccoli florets

Instructions:

1. Preheat oven to 375°F (190°C).

2. Place salmon fillets on a baking sheet lined with foil. Drizzle with olive oil and lemon juice, then sprinkle with paprika, salt, and pepper. Bake for 12-15 minutes or until salmon flakes easily with a fork.

3. In a saucepan, bring water or broth to a boil. Add quinoa, reduce heat, cover, and simmer for 15-20 minutes or until liquid is absorbed.

4. Steam broccoli for 5-7 minutes until tender but crisp.

5. Serve baked salmon alongside cooked quinoa and steamed broccoli.

Turkey and Vegetable Stir-Fry with Brown Rice

Prep/Cooking Time:

25-30 minutes

Nutritional Info: (Per Serving - Turkey Stir-Fry with Rice)

- Calories: 340

- Protein: 30g

- Carbohydrates: 35g

- Fat: 10g

- Fiber: 6g

Ingredients:

- 1 pound lean ground turkey

- 2 tablespoons low-sodium soy sauce

- 1 tablespoon sesame oil

- 2 cloves garlic, minced

- 1 tablespoon grated ginger

- 2 cups mixed vegetables (bell peppers, snap peas, carrots)

- 2 cups cooked brown rice

Instructions:

1. In a skillet over medium heat, cook ground turkey until browned. Add soy sauce, sesame oil, garlic, and ginger. Stir-fry for 2-3 minutes.

2. Add mixed vegetables to the skillet and continue to stir-fry for an additional 5-6 minutes until vegetables are tender yet crisp.

3. Serve the turkey and vegetable stir-fry over cooked brown rice.

Tofu and Veggie Skewers with Quinoa Salad

Prep/Cooking Time:

30-35 minutes

Nutritional Info: (Per Serving - Tofu Skewers with Quinoa Salad)

- Calories: 290

- Protein: 20g

- Carbohydrates: 30g

- Fat: 10g

- Fiber: 6g

Ingredients:

- 1 block firm tofu, pressed and cut into cubes

- 2 tablespoons low-sodium soy sauce

- 1 tablespoon olive oil

- 1 teaspoon smoked paprika

- Assorted vegetables (bell peppers, onions, cherry tomatoes)

- Wooden skewers, soaked in water

- 1 cup cooked quinoa

- 2 tablespoons balsamic vinegar

- 1 tablespoon chopped fresh herbs (parsley, basil)

- Salt and pepper to taste

Instructions:

1. In a bowl, marinate tofu cubes with soy sauce, olive oil, and smoked paprika. Let it sit for 15-20 minutes.

2. Thread marinated tofu cubes and assorted vegetables onto skewers.

3. Preheat grill or grill pan to medium-high heat. Grill skewers for 10-12 minutes, turning occasionally, until tofu is lightly browned and vegetables are tender.

4. In another bowl, mix cooked quinoa with balsamic vinegar, fresh herbs, salt, and pepper to make the salad.

5. Serve tofu and veggie skewers with a side of quinoa salad.

Lean Beef and Mushroom Lettuce Wraps

Prep/Cooking Time:

20-25 minutes

Nutritional Info: (Per Serving - Beef Lettuce Wraps)

- Calories: 280

- Protein: 25g

- Carbohydrates: 10g

- Fat: 15g

- Fiber: 3g

Ingredients:

- 1 pound lean ground beef

- 2 tablespoons low-sodium soy sauce

- 1 tablespoon hoisin sauce

- 2 cloves garlic, minced

- 1 cup mushrooms, finely chopped

- 1 red bell pepper, diced

- 1 head butter lettuce, leaves separated

- Optional toppings: sliced green onions, sesame seeds

Instructions:

1. In a skillet over medium heat, cook ground beef until browned. Add soy sauce, hoisin sauce, garlic, mushrooms, and bell pepper. Stir-fry for 5-7 minutes until vegetables are tender.

2. Spoon the beef and vegetable mixture into individual lettuce leaves.

3. Garnish with sliced green onions and sesame seeds if desired.

Certainly, here are five more unique dinner recipes designed to support muscle growth and fat loss:

Shrimp and Veggie Stir-Fry with Cauliflower Rice

Ingredients:

- 1 pound large shrimp, peeled and deveined

- 2 tablespoons low-sodium soy sauce

- 1 tablespoon sesame oil

- 2 cloves garlic, minced

- 1 tablespoon grated ginger

- 2 cups mixed vegetables (broccoli, bell peppers, snow peas)

- 1 head cauliflower, grated or processed into rice-like texture

- 1 tablespoon olive oil

- Salt and pepper to taste

Instructions:

1. In a bowl, combine shrimp with soy sauce, sesame oil, garlic, and ginger. Let it marinate for 10-15 minutes.

2. Heat olive oil in a skillet over medium-high heat. Stir-fry marinated shrimp for 2-3 minutes until they turn pink. Remove from skillet and set aside.

3. In the same skillet, add more oil if needed and stir-fry mixed vegetables for 5-6 minutes until they're tender-crisp.

4. Add cauliflower rice to the skillet and cook for 3-4 minutes until heated through. Season with salt and pepper.

5. Serve shrimp over the cauliflower rice and vegetable stir-fry.

Prep/Cooking Time:

20-25 minutes

Nutritional Info: (Per Serving - Shrimp Stir-Fry with Cauliflower Rice)

- Calories: 250

- Protein: 30g

- Carbohydrates: 15g

- Fat: 8g

- Fiber: 6g

Baked Chicken Parmesan with Zucchini Noodles

Prep/Cooking Time:

35-40 minutes

Nutritional Info: (Per Serving - Chicken Parmesan with Zucchini Noodles)

- Calories: 320

- Protein: 35g

- Carbohydrates: 20g

- Fat: 10g

- Fiber: 5g

Ingredients:

- 4 boneless, skinless chicken breasts
- 1 cup whole wheat bread crumbs
- ½ cup grated Parmesan cheese
- 1 teaspoon Italian seasoning
- 2 eggs, beaten
- 2 cups marinara sauce
- 4 medium zucchinis, spiralized into noodles
- Cooking spray

Instructions:

1. Preheat oven to 400°F (200°C).

2. In one bowl, mix bread crumbs, Parmesan cheese, and Italian seasoning. Dip each chicken breast in beaten eggs and then coat with the breadcrumb mixture.

3. Place the breaded chicken breasts on a baking sheet sprayed with cooking spray. Bake for 20-25 minutes until cooked through.

4. In a skillet, heat marinara sauce. Add spiralized zucchini noodles and cook for 2-3 minutes until heated through.

5. Serve baked chicken parmesan over zucchini noodles with marinara sauce.

Tuna and Avocado Salad Stuffed Bell Peppers

Prep/Cooking Time:

20-25 minutes

Nutritional Info: (Per Serving - Tuna Avocado Stuffed Peppers)

- Calories: 230

- Protein: 25g

- Carbohydrates: 15g

- Fat: 10g

- Fiber: 6g

Ingredients:

- 4 bell peppers, halved and seeds removed

- 2 cans (5 oz each) tuna, drained

- 1 avocado, diced

- ¼ cup Greek yogurt

- 2 tablespoons lemon juice

- 1 teaspoon Dijon mustard

- Salt and pepper to taste

- Optional: chopped fresh herbs (parsley, cilantro)

Instructions:

1. Preheat oven to 375°F (190°C).

2. In a bowl, mix tuna, diced avocado, Greek yogurt, lemon juice, mustard, salt, pepper, and herbs (if using).

3. Fill each bell pepper half with the tuna and avocado salad mixture.

4. Place stuffed bell peppers on a baking sheet and bake for 15-20 minutes until peppers are tender.

Eggplant and Turkey Lasagna Rolls

Prep/Cooking Time:

40-45 minutes

Nutritional Info: (Per Serving - Eggplant Turkey Lasagna Rolls)

- Calories: 280

- Protein: 30g

- Carbohydrates: 15g

- Fat: 10g

- Fiber: 5g

Ingredients:

- 1 large eggplant, thinly sliced lengthwise

- 1 pound lean ground turkey

- 2 cups marinara sauce

- 1 cup low-fat ricotta cheese

- ½ cup grated mozzarella cheese

- 2 tablespoons chopped fresh basil

- Salt and pepper to taste

Instructions:

1. Preheat oven to 375°F (190°C). Place eggplant slices on a baking sheet, sprinkle with salt, and bake for 8-10 minutes until slightly tender.

2. In a skillet, cook ground turkey until browned. Add marinara sauce and simmer for 5 minutes.

3. In a bowl, mix ricotta cheese, mozzarella cheese, chopped basil, salt, and pepper.

4. Spread a spoonful of the cheese mixture on each eggplant slice, add a spoonful of the turkey mixture, and roll it up.

5. Place the rolled eggplant lasagna in a baking dish, top with remaining marinara sauce, and bake for 20-25 minutes until bubbly and golden.

Black Bean and Chicken Quinoa Bowl

Prep/Cooking Time:*

25-30 minutes

Nutritional Info: (Per Serving - Black Bean Chicken Quinoa Bowl)

- Calories: 320

- Protein: 30g

- Carbohydrates: 30g

- Fat: 10g

- Fiber: 10g

Ingredients:

- 1 cup cooked quinoa

- 1 can (15 oz) black beans, drained and rinsed

- 2 boneless, skinless chicken breasts, grilled and sliced

- 1 avocado, sliced

- 1 cup cherry tomatoes, halved

- ¼ cup chopped cilantro

- Lime wedges for serving

- Optional: salsa, Greek yogurt (as toppings)

Instructions:

1. Divide cooked quinoa among serving bowls.

2. Top with black beans, grilled chicken slices, avocado, cherry tomatoes, and chopped cilantro.

3. Serve with lime wedges for squeezing over the bowl and add optional toppings like salsa or Greek yogurt if desired.

CHAPTER 6: SNACKS AND SIDES

SMART SNACKING

Protein-Packed Turkey Meatballs

Prep and Cooking Time:

30 minutes

Nutritional Info (per serving - about 4 meatballs):

- Calories: 180

- Protein: 24g

- Fat: 8g

- Carbohydrates: 2g

Ingredients:

- 1 pound lean ground turkey

- 1/4 cup almond flour

- 1/4 cup grated Parmesan cheese

- 1 large egg

- 2 cloves garlic, minced

- 2 tablespoons chopped fresh parsley

- Salt and pepper to taste

Instructions:

1. Preheat oven to 375°F (190°C).

2. In a bowl, combine ground turkey, almond flour, Parmesan cheese, egg, garlic, parsley, salt, and pepper. Mix until well combined.

3. Form mixture into small meatballs and place them on a lined baking sheet.

4. Bake for 18-20 minutes until golden brown and cooked through.

Zucchini Noodle Caprese Salad

Prep and Cooking Time:

15 minutes

Nutritional Info (per serving):

- Calories: 120

- Protein: 7g

- Fat: 8g

- Carbohydrates: 8g

Ingredients:

- 2 large zucchinis, spiralized into noodles

- 1 cup cherry tomatoes, halved

- 1/2 cup fresh mozzarella balls

- 2 tablespoons chopped fresh basil

- 2 tablespoons balsamic vinegar

- 1 tablespoon olive oil

- Salt and pepper to taste

Instructions:

1. In a bowl, combine zucchini noodles, cherry tomatoes, mozzarella balls, and basil.

2. In a small bowl, whisk together balsamic vinegar, olive oil, salt, and pepper.

3. Pour the dressing over the salad and toss gently to coat.

Spicy Roasted Chickpeas

Prep and Cooking Time:

40 minutes

Nutritional Info (per serving - about 1/2 cup):

- Calories: 150

- Protein: 6g

- Fat: 5g

- Carbohydrates: 20g

Ingredients:

- 2 cans (15 oz each) chickpeas, drained and rinsed

- 2 tablespoons olive oil

- 1 teaspoon smoked paprika

- 1/2 teaspoon cayenne pepper

- 1/2 teaspoon garlic powder

- Salt to taste

Instructions:

1. Preheat oven to 400°F (200°C).

2. Pat dry the chickpeas using a paper towel to remove excess moisture.

3. In a bowl, toss chickpeas with olive oil, smoked paprika, cayenne pepper, garlic powder, and salt until evenly coated.

4. Spread chickpeas on a baking sheet in a single layer.

5. Roast for 25-30 minutes, shaking the pan occasionally, until crispy.

Cottage Cheese and Veggie Stuffed Bell Peppers

Prep and Cooking Time:

15 minutes

Nutritional Info (per serving - 1 stuffed bell pepper half):

- Calories: 90

- Protein: 7g

- Fat: 1g

- Carbohydrates: 13g

Ingredients:

- 4 bell peppers, halved and deseeded

- 1 cup low-fat cottage cheese

- 1/2 cup diced cucumber

- 1/2 cup diced red onion

- 1/2 cup diced tomatoes

- 2 tablespoons chopped fresh parsley

- Salt and pepper to taste

Instructions:

1. In a bowl, mix together cottage cheese, cucumber, red onion, tomatoes, parsley, salt, and pepper.

2. Spoon the mixture into the halved bell peppers.

3. Refrigerate for at least 30 minutes before serving.

Baked Sweet Potato Fries

Prep and Cooking Time:

40 minutes

Nutritional Info (per serving - about 1 cup):

- Calories: 150

- Protein: 2g

- Fat: 4g

- Carbohydrates: 27g

Ingredients:

- 2 large sweet potatoes, cut into fries

- 1 tablespoon olive oil

- 1 teaspoon smoked paprika

- 1/2 teaspoon garlic powder

- Salt and pepper to taste

Instructions:

1. Preheat oven to 425°F (220°C).

2. In a bowl, toss sweet potato fries with olive oil, smoked paprika, garlic powder, salt, and pepper until evenly coated.

3. Spread fries on a baking sheet in a single layer.

4. Bake for 25-30 minutes, flipping halfway through, until crispy.

Greek Yogurt and Berry Parfait

Prep Time:

5 minutes

Nutritional Info (per serving):

- Calories: 200

- Protein: 18g

- Fat: 4g

- Carbohydrates: 25g

Ingredients:

- 1 cup Greek yogurt (plain or flavored)

- 1/2 cup mixed berries (strawberries, blueberries, raspberries)

- 2 tablespoons granola

- 1 tablespoon honey (optional)

Instructions:

1. In a glass or jar, layer Greek yogurt, mixed berries, and granola.

2. Drizzle honey on top for added sweetness if desired.

3. Repeat the layers until the container is filled.

Quinoa and Black Bean Salad

Prep Time:

15 minutes

Nutritional Info (per serving):

- Calories: 220

- Protein: 9g

- Fat: 7g

- Carbohydrates: 32g

Ingredients:

- 1 cup cooked quinoa

- 1 can (15 oz) black beans, drained and rinsed

- 1 red bell pepper, diced

- 1/2 cup corn kernels (fresh, frozen, or canned)

- 1/4 cup chopped fresh cilantro

- Juice of 1 lime

- 2 tablespoons olive oil

- Salt and pepper to taste

Instructions:

1. In a large bowl, combine cooked quinoa, black beans, diced bell pepper, corn kernels, and cilantro.

2. In a separate small bowl, whisk together lime juice, olive oil, salt, and pepper.

3. Pour the dressing over the salad and toss gently to combine.

Tuna Stuffed Cucumber Boats

Prep Time:

10 minutes

Nutritional Info (per serving - 2 stuffed cucumber halves):

- Calories: 140

- Protein: 18g

- Fat: 3g

- Carbohydrates: 11g

Ingredients:

- 2 large cucumbers

- 1 can (5 oz) tuna, drained

- 1/4 cup plain Greek yogurt

- 2 tablespoons finely chopped red onion

- 1 tablespoon chopped dill or parsley

- Salt and pepper to taste

Instructions:

1. Cut cucumbers in half lengthwise and scoop out the seeds to create a hollow center.

2. In a bowl, mix together drained tuna, Greek yogurt, red onion, dill or parsley, salt, and pepper.

3. Spoon the tuna mixture into the hollowed-out cucumbers.

Edamame and Avocado Dip with Veggie Sticks

Prep Time:

10 minutes

Nutritional Info (per serving - 2 tablespoons dip with veggies):

- Calories: 70

- Protein: 3g

- Fat: 5g

- Carbohydrates: 5g

Ingredients:

- 1 cup shelled edamame, cooked and cooled

- 1 ripe avocado

- 2 tablespoons lime juice

- 1 clove garlic, minced

- Salt and pepper to taste

- Assorted veggie sticks (carrots, celery, bell peppers) for dipping

Instructions:

1. In a food processor, combine cooked edamame, avocado, lime juice, garlic, salt, and pepper. Blend until smooth.

2. Serve the dip with assorted veggie sticks for dipping.

Cauliflower Buffalo Bites

Prep and Cooking Time:

30 minutes

Nutritional Info (per serving - about 1 cup):

- Calories: 80

- Protein: 3g

- Fat: 6g

- Carbohydrates: 5g

Ingredients:

- 1 head cauliflower, cut into florets

- 1/2 cup buffalo sauce

- 2 tablespoons olive oil

- 1 teaspoon garlic powder

- Ranch or blue cheese dressing for dipping (optional)

Instructions:

1. Preheat oven to 450°F (230°C).

2. In a bowl, toss cauliflower florets with buffalo sauce, olive oil, and garlic powder until coated.

3. Spread cauliflower on a baking sheet lined with parchment paper.

4. Bake for 20-25 minutes, until cauliflower is crispy.

CHAPTER 7 : DESSERTS AND TREATS

GUILT-FREE SWEET INDULGENCES

Protein-Packed Chocolate Avocado Mousse

Prep & Cooking Time:

- Prep Time: 10 minutes

- Cooking Time: 0 minutes

- Total Time: 1 hour 10 minutes (including chilling)

Nutritional Info (per serving):

- Calories: 180

- Protein: 8g

- Fat: 10g

- Carbohydrates: 20g

- Fiber: 6g

- Sugar: 10g

Ingredients:

- 2 ripe avocados

- 1/4 cup unsweetened cocoa powder

- 1/4 cup almond milk

- 1/4 cup honey or maple syrup

- 2 scoops chocolate protein powder

- 1 teaspoon vanilla extract

- Pinch of salt

Instructions:

1. In a food processor, blend avocados until smooth.

2. Add cocoa powder, almond milk, honey/maple syrup, protein powder, vanilla extract, and salt. Blend until well combined.

3. Taste and adjust sweetness if needed by adding more sweetener.

4. Divide into serving cups and refrigerate for at least 1 hour before serving.

Berry Protein Popsicles

Prep & Cooking Time:

- Prep Time: 10 minutes

- Cooking Time: 0 minutes

- Total Time: 4 hours 10 minutes

Nutritional Info (per serving):

- Calories: 90

- Protein: 10g

- Fat: 1g

- Carbohydrates: 10g

- Fiber: 2g

- Sugar: 7g

Ingredients:

- 1 cup mixed berries (strawberries, blueberries, raspberries)
- 1 cup Greek yogurt
- 2 scoops vanilla protein powder
- 1 tablespoon honey or sweetener of choice

Instructions:

1. Blend mixed berries until smooth.

2. In a separate bowl, mix Greek yogurt, protein powder, and honey/sweetener.

3. Layer the berry puree and yogurt mixture into popsicle molds.

4. Insert popsicle sticks and freeze for at least 4 hours or until solid.

Protein Peanut Butter Cookies

Prep & Cooking Time:

- Prep Time: 15 minutes
- Cooking Time: 10-12 minutes
- Total Time: 27-29 minutes

Nutritional Info (per serving, 2 cookies):

- Calories: 180
- Protein: 10g

- Fat: 12g

- Carbohydrates: 12g

- Fiber: 2g

- Sugar: 7g

Ingredients:

- 1 cup natural peanut butter

- 1/4 cup honey or maple syrup

- 1 egg

- 1 teaspoon vanilla extract

- 2 scoops vanilla protein powder

- 1/2 teaspoon baking soda

Instructions:

1. Preheat oven to 350°F (175°C) and line a baking sheet with parchment paper.

2. In a bowl, mix peanut butter, honey/maple syrup, egg, and vanilla extract until smooth.

3. Add protein powder and baking soda, mix until combined.

4. Roll dough into small balls, place on the baking sheet, and press down gently with a fork.

5. Bake for 10-12 minutes until edges are golden brown.

6. Allow to cool before serving.

Chocolate Protein Bars

Prep & Cooking Time:

- Prep Time: 10 minutes

- Cooking Time: 0 minutes

- Total Time: 1-2 hours 10 minutes

Nutritional Info (per serving, 1 bar):

- Calories: 180

- Protein: 10g

- Fat: 8g

- Carbohydrates: 20g

- Fiber: 4g

- Sugar: 8g

Ingredients:

- 1 cup rolled oats

- 1/2 cup almond butter

- 1/4 cup honey or maple syrup

- 2 scoops chocolate protein powder

- 1/4 cup unsweetened cocoa powder

- 1/4 cup almond milk

Instructions:

1. In a bowl, mix rolled oats, almond butter, honey/maple syrup, protein powder, and cocoa powder.

2. Slowly add almond milk until the mixture sticks together.

3. Press the mixture into a lined baking dish and refrigerate for 1-2 hours.

4. Cut into bars and store in the refrigerator.

Protein-Packed Chia Seed Pudding

Prep & Cooking Time:

- Prep Time: 5 minutes

- Cooking Time: 0 minutes

- Total Time: 2 hours 5 minutes (including chilling)

Nutritional Info (per serving):

- Calories: 170

- Protein: 10g

- Fat: 7g

- Carbohydrates: 15g

- Fiber: 10g

- Sugar: 5g

Ingredients:

- 1/4 cup chia seeds

- 1 cup almond milk

- 1 scoop vanilla protein powder

- 1 tablespoon honey or maple syrup

- Fresh fruit for topping (optional)

Instructions:

1. In a bowl, mix chia seeds, almond milk, protein powder, and sweetener.

2. Stir well and refrigerate for at least 2 hours or overnight, stirring occasionally until it thickens.

3. Serve chilled with fresh fruit toppings if desired.

CHAPTER 8 : MEAL PLANS AND SAMPLE MENUS

CUSTOMIZABLE MEAL PLANS FOR MUSCLE GAIN

Day 1:

- **Breakfast:** Protein-Packed Peanut Butter Banana Ice Cream

- **Lunch:** High-Protein Berry Parfait

- **Dinner:** Protein-Packed Chocolate Avocado Mousse

Day 2:

- **Breakfast:** High-Protein Berry Parfait

- **Lunch:** Protein-Rich Chia Seed Pudding

- **Dinner:** Low-Calorie Protein Brownies

Day 3:

- **Breakfast:** Low-Calorie Protein Brownies

- **Lunch:** Protein-Packed Peanut Butter Banana Ice Cream

- **Dinner:** High-Protein Berry Parfait

Day 4:

- **Breakfast:** Protein-Rich Chia Seed Pudding

- **Lunch:** Low-Calorie Protein Brownies

- **Dinner:** Protein-Packed Chocolate Avocado Mousse

Day 5:

- **Breakfast:** Protein-Packed Chocolate Avocado Mousse
- **Lunch:** High-Protein Berry Parfait
- **Dinner:** Protein-Rich Chia Seed Pudding

Day 6:

- **Breakfast:** High-Protein Berry Parfait
- **Lunch:** Protein-Packed Chocolate Avocado Mousse
- **Dinner:** Low-Calorie Protein Brownies

Day 7:

- **Breakfast:** Low-Calorie Protein Brownies
- **Lunch:** Protein-Rich Chia Seed Pudding
- **Dinner:** Protein-Packed Peanut Butter Banana Ice Cream

- **Preparation:** Prep your meals in advance for the week to ensure consistency.
- **Portion Control:** Adjust portion sizes based on your caloric and protein intake goals.
- **Fluid Intake:** Stay hydrated throughout the day, aiming for at least 8 glasses of water.
- **Exercise:** Complement your meal plan with a well-structured workout routine focusing on resistance training to aid muscle growth.

TAILORING MEAL PLANS TO INDIVIDUAL NEEDS

Customizing meal plans based on individual needs is paramount for optimizing nutrition, achieving fitness goals, and ensuring sustainability. When aiming for muscle gain, personalizing your meal plan involves considering various factors:

1. Caloric Needs: Everyone has different calorie requirements based on factors like age, weight, height, activity level, and metabolism. Calculate your Total Daily Energy Expenditure (TDEE) and adjust your meal plan to meet your specific caloric needs for muscle growth.

2. Macro-nutrient Balance: Customize the ratio of macro-nutrients (proteins, carbohydrates, and fats) in your meals according to your body's response. For muscle gain, prioritize protein intake to support muscle repair and growth, while balancing carbohydrates for energy and fats for overall health.

3. Meal Timing: Tailor meal timing based on your daily schedule and workout routine. Consider consuming a higher proportion of carbohydrates and protein around workouts to support energy levels and muscle recovery.

4. Food Preferences and Allergies: Adapt recipes and ingredients based on personal preferences and dietary restrictions. Substitute ingredients in recipes to accommodate allergies or intolerances without compromising nutritional content.

5. Portion Control: While the provided meal plan offers variety, adjust portion sizes based on individual needs and goals. Portion control ensures you're consuming adequate nutrients without exceeding calorie requirements.

6. Monitoring Progress: Regularly track progress by assessing body composition changes, strength gains, and energy levels. Adjust the meal plan as needed based on the observed outcomes and any changes in goals.

7. Hydration: Remember the significance of staying hydrated. Adequate water intake is essential for overall health, digestion, and optimal muscle function.

8. Consultation and Adaptation: Seek guidance from a nutritionist, dietitian, or fitness professional to personalize your meal plan further. They can offer expert advice, considering your specific goals, lifestyle, and any underlying health conditions.

Remember, the provided meal plan is a starting point. Adjustments should be made based on individual responses, ensuring the meal plan supports your unique journey towards muscle gain while promoting overall health and well-being.

CHAPTER 9 : TIPS FOR SUCCESS AND SUSTAINABILITY

STAYING MOTIVATED ON THE JOURNEY

1. Set Realistic Goals: Define achievable and realistic goals. Break them down into smaller milestones, making them more manageable and allowing you to celebrate progress along the way.

2. Create a Balanced Plan: Develop a balanced and flexible meal plan that suits your lifestyle. Incorporate a variety of foods you enjoy, including healthy options that support your goals.

3. Prioritize Sustainability: Avoid drastic, short-term approaches. Instead, focus on sustainable habits that you can maintain over time. Consistency over perfection is key.

4. Monitor Progress: Keep track of your progress through journaling, measurements, or photos. Seeing positive changes can be a great motivator and help you stay on track.

5. Find Support: Surround yourself with supportive friends, family, or a community that shares your health goals. Their encouragement and shared experiences can keep you motivated.

6. Embrace Flexibility: Understand that setbacks or deviations from your plan are normal. Learn from these experiences and use them as opportunities to adjust and continue moving forward.

7. Celebrate Achievements: Celebrate your achievements, no matter how small. Acknowledging your progress can boost motivation and reinforce positive behaviors.

8. Keep Learning: Educate yourself about nutrition, fitness, and overall health. The more you understand about your body and its needs, the better equipped you'll be to make informed choices.

9. Practice Self-Compassion: Be kind to yourself throughout the journey. Don't be too hard on yourself for occasional slip-ups. Treat yourself with compassion and get back on track.

10. Focus on Non-Scale Victories: Recognize achievements beyond the number on the scale. Improved energy levels, better sleep, or increased strength are equally important markers of progress.

11. Stay Consistent: Consistency is key to success. Even on challenging days, stick to your plan as closely as possible to maintain momentum.

12. Revisit and Adjust: Regularly reassess your goals and approach. Adjustments may be necessary as your body adapts or your circumstances change.

Remember, the journey towards improved health and fitness is not just about reaching a destination; it's about embracing a lifestyle that promotes well-being in the long run. Stay patient, stay consistent, and embrace the journey, knowing that each step forward is a step closer to your goals.

CONCLUSION

Throughout these pages, we've explored the art of crafting delicious meals that not only fuel the body but also align with specific goals—whether it's sculpting lean muscle or shedding excess weight. The recipes presented here, meticulously designed to be high in protein yet low in calories, serve as a testament to the idea that taste need not be sacrificed for health.

But this book is more than just a collection of recipes; it's a roadmap toward sustainable wellness. It's about empowering you to take charge of your dietary habits, encouraging thoughtful meal preparation, and fostering a deeper understanding of the profound connection between food and the body's transformation.

As you journey through this cookbook, may you find inspiration in the kitchen, discovering the joy of preparing nourishing meals that energize and support your body's needs. May you embrace the principles of balance, consistency, and self-care, recognizing that every meal is an opportunity to nourish not only your physical being but also your aspirations for a healthier, more vibrant life.

Remember, the recipes within these pages are not just ingredients and instructions; they represent a commitment—to your well-being, to your goals, and to the belief that small, deliberate choices made every day can lead to monumental changes over time.

As you close this cookbook, may the flavors linger on your palate, the lessons linger in your mind, and may your journey towards a healthier, stronger, and more vibrant you continue, one delicious meal at a time.

APPENDIX

METRIC CONVERSION CHART

Volume Conversions

- 1 teaspoon (tsp) = 5 milliliters (ml)

- 1 tablespoon (tbsp) = 15 milliliters (ml)

- 1 fluid ounce (fl oz) = 30 milliliters (ml)

- 1 cup = 240 milliliters (ml)

- 1 pint (pt) = 480 milliliters (ml)

- 1 quart (qt) = 0.95 liters (l)

- 1 gallon (gal) = 3.8 liters (l)

Weight Conversions (Dry Ingredients)

- 1 ounce (oz) = 28 grams (g)

- 1 pound (lb) = 454 grams (g)

- 1 kilogram (kg) = 1000 grams (g)

Temperature Conversions

- Celsius to Fahrenheit: $F = C \times 9/5 + 32$

  - 0°C = 32°F

  - 100°C = 212°F

- Fahrenheit to Celsius: $C = (F - 32) \times 5/9$

  - 32°F = 0°C

  - 212°F = 100°C

Length Conversions

- 1 inch (in) = 2.54 centimeters (cm)

- 1 foot (ft) = 30.48 centimeters (cm)

- 1 yard (yd) = 0.91 meters (m)

- 1 mile = 1.61 kilometers (km)

Oven Temperature Equivalents

- Low heat: 120°C - 150°C (250°F - 300°F)

- Moderate heat: 160°C - 180°C (325°F - 350°F)

- Moderate to high heat: 190°C - 230°C (375°F - 450°F)

- High heat: 240°C - 260°C (475°F - 500°F)

Common Kitchen Measurements

- 1 stick of butter = 113 grams (g) = 1/2 cup

- 1 liter of water = approximately 4 cups

- 1 kilogram of flour = approximately 8 cups

- 1 medium egg = approximately 50 grams (g)

Oven Racks Position

- Top rack: Generally for broiling or to brown the tops of dishes.

- Middle rack: For most baking and roasting.

- Bottom rack: Used for crisping crusts or cooking foods that require a lower temperature.

Liquid Measurements for Precision

- Use a liquid measuring cup for accurate volume measurements.

- Fill to the appropriate line by looking at the measurement at eye level.

INGREDIENT SUBSTITUITION GUIDE

In the journey towards healthier eating, flexibility in the kitchen can be your greatest ally. Understanding ingredient substitutions not only empowers you to adapt recipes to suit your dietary preferences but also allows for creative experimentation without compromising flavor or nutrition.

Here are some useful tips for ingredient substitution:

1. Sweeteners:

- **Natural Alternatives:** Replace refined sugars with healthier options like honey, maple syrup, or stevia for sweetness.

- **Fruit Purees:** Use mashed bananas or unsweetened applesauce in baking to reduce added sugars.

2. Fats:

-**Healthy Oils:** Opt for olive oil, avocado oil, or coconut oil instead of butter or margarine for a healthier fat profile.

- **Greek Yogurt:** Substitute part of the oil or butter in recipes with Greek yogurt for moisture and richness.

3. Flours and Grains:

- **Whole Grains:** Replace refined flours with whole wheat flour, almond flour, or oat flour for added fiber and nutrients.

- **Gluten-Free Options:** Experiment with gluten-free alternatives like rice flour, quinoa flour, or chickpea flour.

4. Dairy:

- **Plant-Based Milks:** Swap cow's milk with almond, soy, or oat milk for lactose-free and lower-calorie options.

- **Nutritional Yeast:** Use nutritional yeast as a cheesy substitute in recipes calling for cheese.

5. Proteins:

- **Plant-Based Proteins:** Incorporate tofu, tempeh, or legumes like beans and lentils as alternatives to meat for a lighter protein source.

- **Lean Meats:** Choose lean cuts of meat like skinless chicken or turkey for lower fat content.

6. Seasonings and Flavor Enhancers:

- **Herbs and Spices:** Experiment with fresh herbs and spices to add flavor without relying on excessive salt or seasoning blends.

Remember, while substitutions can often elevate the nutritional value of a dish, it's essential to consider the taste and texture changes that may occur. Feel free to tweak and adjust recipes to your liking, allowing your creativity to flourish in the kitchen while supporting your health and wellness goals.

Thank you

for embarking on this culinary journey. We hope these recipes have tantalized your taste buds and sparked joy in your kitchen.

If you've enjoyed the flavors within these pages, **we kindly ask you to share your thoughts and experiences by KINDLY leaving a review.** Your feedback means the world to us and helps others discover the delights awaiting them in this cookbook.

Happy cooking, and may your kitchen always be filled with laughter and delicious aromas!

www.ingramcontent.com/pod-product-compliance
Lightning Source LLC
Chambersburg PA
CBHW071608270726
48661CB00019B/1658